ENDOMORPH

DIET AND FOOD LIST FOR SENIORS

Ultimate Guide and Exercise to Boost your Metabolism and lose weight with Delicious Recipes

Dr. JANE THORNTHWAITE

TABLE OF CONTENTS

Chapter One

INTRODUCTION

What is an endomorph body type?

Endomorph is one of the three fundamental body types, as proposed by American psychologist William Sheldon. Individuals with an endomorph body type are generally characterized by a softer, rounder body shape, featuring a higher percentage of body fat, particularly in the lower body regions such as the hips, thighs, and buttocks. Endomorphs typically possess a slower metabolism, making weight gain easier and weight loss more challenging for them.

Common physical attributes associated with the endomorph body type include a broad, round, and soft physique, shorter limbs, a wider waistline, and a tendency to store excess fat in the lower body. Endomorphs often exhibit a more relaxed, easy-going personality and tend to adopt a laid-back approach to life.

While some individuals may inherently have an endomorph body type, it is crucial to recognize that body type does not conclusively determine one's health or fitness. Through proper diet, exercise, and lifestyle habits, individuals of all body types can attain a healthy and active lifestyle.

Why is diet and exercise important for seniors with endomorph body type?

Diet and exercise are important for seniors with an endomorph body type for several reasons. As people age, their metabolism tends to slow down, and they may become more prone to weight gain and other health issues. Endomorphs already have a slower metabolism, which can make it even more challenging to maintain a healthy weight as they age.

Here are some reasons why diet and exercise are particularly important for seniors with an endomorph body type:

• Weight management: Endomorphs tend to gain weight more easily than other body types. Regular exercise and a healthy diet can help seniors with an endomorph body type manage their weight and maintain healthy body composition.

• Reduced risk of chronic diseases: A healthy diet and regular exercise can help prevent or manage chronic diseases, such as heart disease, diabetes, and high blood pressure, which are more common in seniors.

• Improved mobility and balance: Endomorphs often carry more weight in their lower body, which can put additional stress on their joints and make it harder to maintain balance. Regular exercise can help improve mobility, balance, and overall physical function.

•   Enhanced mental health: Exercise and a healthy diet have been shown to improve mood and reduce symptoms of depression and anxiety, which are common among seniors.

Overall, a healthy diet and regular exercise are crucial for seniors with an endomorph body type to maintain good health and quality of life as they age. It's important to consult with a healthcare professional and a certified fitness trainer to develop an appropriate exercise and nutrition plan based on individual needs and limitations.

Benefits of proper diet and exercise for seniors

Proper diet and exercise play crucial roles in the well-being of seniors for a variety of reasons. As individuals age, their bodies undergo changes that heighten the risk of health issues and limit mobility. Nonetheless, maintaining a routine of regular exercise and adhering to a healthy diet can assist seniors in preserving both their physical and mental health, ultimately enhancing their overall quality of life.

The following are some benefits associated with proper diet and exercise for seniors:

- **Improved cardiovascular health:** Regular exercise contributes to enhanced heart health by fortifying the heart muscle, lowering blood pressure, and promoting better blood circulation. A healthy diet further aids in managing cholesterol levels, reducing the likelihood of heart disease.

- **Stronger bones and muscles:** Exercise, particularly weight-bearing activities, helps boost bone density and muscle strength, thereby diminishing the risk of falls and fractures among seniors.

- **Increased mobility and flexibility:** Regular exercise aids in the maintenance of seniors' mobility and flexibility, facilitating the performance of daily activities and lowering the risk of injury.

- **Improved mental health:** Exercise and a nutritious diet have demonstrated positive effects on mood, stress reduction, anxiety alleviation, and the prevention of cognitive decline in seniors.

- **Reduced risk of chronic diseases:** Adhering to a healthy diet and engaging in regular exercise can serve as preventive measures or management strategies for chronic diseases, including diabetes, osteoporosis, and certain forms of cancer.

- **Increased social interaction:** Participation in group exercise classes or other physical activities offers seniors opportunities for social engagement, helping reduce feelings of isolation and loneliness.

Chapter Two

UNDERSTANDING ENDOMORPH DIET

What is an endomorph diet?

An endomorph diet is a dietary approach that is designed to support the needs of individuals with an endomorph body type. The endomorph body type is characterized by a higher percentage of body fat, particularly in the lower body, and a slower metabolism. Therefore, the endomorph diet typically focuses on reducing calorie intake while providing a balanced macronutrient ratio to help support weight loss and body composition goals.

Here are some key features of an endomorph diet:

• Focus on protein: Endomorphs tend to have a slower metabolism, and a higher protein intake can help support muscle growth and repair, which can increase metabolic rate. Good sources of protein include lean meats, fish, eggs, dairy, legumes, and tofu.

• Limit carbohydrate intake: Endomorphs tend to be more sensitive to carbohydrates, which can lead to weight gain. The endomorph diet typically emphasizes complex carbohydrates, such as whole grains, fruits, and vegetables, while limiting simple carbohydrates, such as sugar and refined grains.

• Moderate fat intake: A moderate intake of healthy fats can help support satiety and hormone production. Good sources of healthy fats include avocados, nuts, seeds, olive oil, and fatty fish.

- Control portion sizes: Endomorphs may need to eat smaller, more frequent meals to help support their metabolism and manage hunger. Controlling portion sizes and eating on a regular schedule can help support weight loss and body composition goals.

- Drink plenty of water: Staying hydrated is important for overall health and weight loss. Drinking plenty of water can help support digestion, reduce hunger, and improve energy levels.

It's important to note that the endomorph diet is not a one-size-fits-all approach, and individual needs and preferences may vary. Consulting with a registered dietitian or a healthcare professional can help develop a personalized nutrition plan based on individual goals and needs.

Characteristics of endomorph diet

Endomorphs are characterized by a softer, rounder body type and a slower metabolism, making weight loss and maintenance more challenging. In terms of nutrition, endomorphs may find a diet higher in protein and lower in carbohydrates and fats beneficial.

The key characteristics of an endomorph diet include:

High Protein: Endomorphs benefit from a diet rich in protein, aiding in muscle mass development and maintenance, subsequently boosting metabolism. Good protein sources include lean meats, fish, eggs, beans, and low-fat dairy products.

Low Carbohydrate: A lower carbohydrate intake may help endomorphs control blood sugar levels and reduce the risk of weight gain. Recommended carbohydrate sources encompass fruits, vegetables, whole grains, and legumes.

Low Fat: A diet lower in fat can assist endomorphs in reducing overall calorie intake and promoting weight loss. Healthy fat sources include nuts, seeds, avocados, and olive oil.

Portion Control: Due to a slower metabolism and a propensity for weight gain, endomorphs benefit from mindful portion control. Consuming smaller, frequent meals throughout the day helps curb hunger and prevents overeating.

Hydration: Staying hydrated is advantageous for endomorphs, as it aids in appetite control and supports weight loss. Opting for water over sugary beverages maintains proper hydration and promotes overall health.

Exercise: Alongside a nutritious diet, regular exercise is crucial for endomorphs. A combination of strength training and cardiovascular exercise contributes to muscle mass development, metabolism boost, and enhanced overall health, facilitating greater weight loss.

Health hazard related to endomorph body type

Endomorph body type is not necessarily a health hazard in itself, but it can be associated with certain health risks. Endomorphs tend to have higher levels of body fat, particularly in the abdominal area, which can increase the risk of several health conditions, including:

• Type 2 Diabetes: Endomorphs are at a higher risk of developing type 2 diabetes due to the higher levels of body fat, particularly in the abdominal area. This is because excess body fat can impair the body's ability to use insulin effectively, leading to insulin resistance and high blood sugar levels.

•   Cardiovascular Disease: Endomorphs are also at a higher risk of developing cardiovascular disease, which includes conditions such as high blood pressure, high cholesterol, and heart disease. This is because excess body fat can lead to the buildup of plaque in the arteries, increasing the risk of heart attack and stroke.

•   Sleep Apnea: Endomorphs may also be at a higher risk of developing sleep apnea, which is a condition where breathing is interrupted during sleep. This is because excess body fat can cause the airways to become blocked during sleep, leading to breathing difficulties and interrupted sleep.

• Joint Pain: Endomorphs may be more prone to joint pain, particularly in the knees and hips, due to the excess weight putting pressure on the joints.

Endomorphs need to maintain a healthy lifestyle by following a balanced diet, engaging in regular physical activity, and managing stress levels to reduce the risk of developing these health conditions.

Chapter Three

ENDOMORPH BODY TYPE EXERCISE FOR SENIORS

Importance of exercise for seniors

Exercise holds significance for seniors due to various reasons, including:

Maintaining Physical Health: Regular exercise aids seniors in preserving physical health by enhancing muscle strength, flexibility, and balance. This, in turn, lowers the risk of falls and injuries, enhances cardiovascular health, and reduces the likelihood of chronic diseases like heart disease and diabetes.

Improving Mental Health: Exercise positively impacts mental health by alleviating symptoms of depression and anxiety, fostering an enhanced mood, and improving overall well-being.

Social Interaction: Engaging in exercise provides seniors with opportunities for social interaction, aiding in the maintenance of connections with others and alleviating feelings of isolation and loneliness.

Cognitive Function: Regular exercise is associated with enhanced cognitive function, encompassing improvements in memory and learning.

Quality of Life: By promoting independence, boosting energy levels, and enhancing both physical and mental health, regular exercise contributes to an overall improvement in the quality of life for seniors.

Seniors should partake in regular exercise, and consultation with a healthcare professional is essential to ensure that the chosen exercise regimen aligns with their fitness level and accommodates any underlying medical conditions safely.

Benefits of regular exercise

Regular exercise provides a multitude of benefits for both physical and mental health.

Here are some of the key benefits of regular exercise:

• Improved cardiovascular health: Exercise helps to strengthen the heart and circulatory system, reducing the risk of heart disease, stroke, and other cardiovascular conditions.

• Weight management: Exercise helps to burn calories and build muscle mass, aiding in weight management and reducing the risk of obesity and related conditions.

- Increased muscle strength and flexibility: Regular exercise can improve muscle strength, flexibility, and endurance, helping to prevent age-related decline in physical function.
- Improved bone density: Weight-bearing exercise helps to improve bone density, reducing the risk of osteoporosis and related conditions.
- Reduced risk of chronic diseases: Exercise has been shown to reduce the risk of chronic conditions such as type 2 diabetes, high blood pressure, and some types of cancer.
- Improved mental health: Exercise releases endorphins, which can help to improve mood and reduce stress, anxiety, and depression.
- Improved cognitive function: Exercise has been linked to improved cognitive

function, including better memory, attention, and problem-solving skills.

• Improved sleep: Exercise can help to regulate sleep patterns, leading to better quality sleep and improved overall health.

Overall, regular exercise is essential for maintaining physical and mental health throughout life, especially as we age.

Challenges faced by seniors with endomorphic body type during exercise

Seniors with an endomorphic body type may encounter several challenges during exercise due to their inherent physique, including:

Difficulty Losing Weight: The slower metabolism and a predisposition to fat storage associated with endomorphic body types can present obstacles to weight loss, making it a more challenging endeavor.

Joint Pain: Those with endomorphic body types might be more susceptible to joint pain and arthritis, potentially intensifying the difficulty and discomfort experienced during exercise.

Reduced Mobility: The larger body size characteristic of endomorphic body types can lead to diminished mobility, rendering certain exercises more strenuous or uncomfortable.

Cardiovascular Strain: The presence of excess weight may impose additional strain on the cardiovascular system, heightening the difficulty of specific exercises and potentially posing risks to overall cardiovascular health.

Risk of Injury: Seniors with an endomorphic body type may contend with weaker muscles and reduced flexibility, elevating their vulnerability to exercise-related injuries.

Types of exercises suitable for endomorphic body type seniors

Endomorphic body type seniors can benefit from a variety of exercises, including:

• Strength training: Resistance training is particularly beneficial for endomorphic body type seniors as it helps to build muscle mass, which can boost metabolism and aid in weight management. Examples of strength training exercises include bodyweight exercises like squats, lunges, push-ups, and planks, as well as exercises with free weights, resistance bands, or weight machines.

• Cardiovascular exercise: Cardiovascular exercise is important for heart health and weight management. Low-impact exercises such as walking, cycling, swimming, and water aerobics are suitable for endomorphic body type seniors as they reduce the risk of joint pain and injury.

• Flexibility and balance training: Flexibility and balance training are important for maintaining mobility and reducing the risk of falls. Endomorphic body type seniors can benefit from exercises such as yoga, tai chi, or Pilates, which focus on stretching, balance, and core strength.

• Low-impact sports: Sports like golf, pickleball, and bocce ball are low-impact and can provide a fun and social way to stay active.

It's important to start gradually and progress slowly with any exercise program to avoid injury and ensure a sustainable routine. Working with a certified fitness trainer or physical therapist can help endomorphic body type seniors design a safe and effective exercise program tailored to their individual needs and abilities.

Chapter Four

EXERCISE FOR ENDOMORPH SENIORS

Why exercise is important for endomorph seniors?

• Weight management: Endomorph seniors tend to have a slower metabolism and a tendency to store fat, making weight management more challenging. Exercise can help to boost metabolism, burn calories, and build muscle mass, which can aid in weight management and improve overall health.

• Improved cardiovascular health: Regular exercise helps to strengthen the heart and circulatory system, reducing the risk of heart disease, stroke, and other cardiovascular conditions.

•	Improved muscle strength and flexibility: Exercise helps to improve muscle strength, flexibility, and endurance, reducing the risk of age-related decline in physical function.

•	Improved bone density: Weight-bearing exercise helps to improve bone density, reducing the risk of osteoporosis and related conditions.

•	Reduced risk of chronic diseases: Exercise has been shown to reduce the risk of chronic conditions such as type 2 diabetes, high blood pressure, and some types of cancer.

•	Improved mental health: Exercise releases endorphins, which can help to improve mood and reduce stress, anxiety, and depression.

• Improved cognitive function: Exercise has been linked to improved cognitive function, including better memory, attention, and problem-solving skills.

• Improved sleep: Exercise can help to regulate sleep patterns, leading to better quality sleep and improved overall health.

Best exercises for endomorph seniors

Endomorph seniors can benefit from a variety of exercises, including:

• Low-impact cardio exercises: Endomorph seniors can benefit from low-impact cardio exercises that are easy on the joints such as walking, swimming, cycling, water aerobics, or using an elliptical machine. These exercises can help to burn calories, boost metabolism, and improve cardiovascular health.

- Strength training exercises: Strength training exercises can help endomorph seniors build muscle mass, which can boost metabolism and aid in weight management. Bodyweight exercises like squats, lunges, push-ups, and planks, as well as exercises with free weights, resistance bands, or weight machines, can be suitable for endomorph seniors.

- Flexibility and balance exercises: Endomorph seniors can benefit from exercises that improve flexibility and balance such as yoga, Pilates, and Tai Chi. These exercises can help to reduce the risk of falls and improve overall mobility.

- Low-impact sports: Endomorph seniors can also participate in low-impact sports such as golf, pickleball, or bocce ball, which provide a fun and social way to stay active.

Endomorph seniors need to start gradually and progress slowly with any exercise program to avoid injury and ensure a sustainable routine.

Resistance training for endomorph seniors

Resistance training, also known as strength training, is an excellent exercise option for endomorph seniors. Resistance training involves using resistance to build muscle strength, improve bone density, and boost metabolism.

Here are some key tips for resistance training for endomorph seniors:

• Start gradually: It's essential to start with light weights or resistance bands and gradually increase the intensity, weight, or resistance over time.

•   Focus on form: Proper form is crucial to avoid injury and get the most benefit from resistance training. Seniors should work with a certified fitness trainer to ensure proper form and technique.

•   Train all major muscle groups: Resistance training should target all major muscle groups, including the arms, chest, back, legs, and core.

•   Use a variety of exercises: Using a variety of exercises can help to prevent boredom and target different muscle groups. Some examples of resistance exercises include bicep curls, tricep extensions, chest presses, leg presses, squats, and lunges.

•   Allow for adequate rest and recovery: Rest is essential for muscle recovery and growth. Seniors should avoid overtraining and allow for adequate rest between resistance training sessions.

•	Incorporate resistance training into a well-rounded exercise program: Resistance training should be part of a well-rounded exercise program that includes cardio, flexibility, and balance exercises.

In conclusion, resistance training can be a safe and effective exercise option for endomorph seniors when done correctly.

Cardiovascular exercise for endomorph seniors

Cardiovascular exercise, also known as cardio, is an essential component of any exercise program, especially for endomorph seniors. Cardio exercises increase the heart rate, improve lung capacity, burn calories, and strengthen the cardiovascular system.

Here are some key tips for cardiovascular exercise for endomorph seniors:

•	Start gradually: It's essential to start with low-intensity cardio exercises and gradually increase the intensity, duration, and frequency over time. Walking, swimming, and cycling are great low-intensity cardio options for endomorph seniors.

•	Choose low-impact exercises: Endomorph seniors should choose low-impact exercises that are easy on the joints to avoid injury. Water aerobics, using an elliptical machine, or using a stationary bike are good options.

•	Monitor heart rate: Endomorph seniors should monitor their heart rate during cardio exercises to ensure they're working at a safe and effective level. A target heart rate range can be calculated based on age and fitness level.

•	Mix it up: Variety is essential to avoid boredom and challenge the cardiovascular system in different ways. Endomorph seniors should mix up their cardio exercises with different types, such as walking one day and swimming the next.

•	Incorporate interval training: Interval training involves alternating between periods of high-intensity exercise and rest or low-intensity exercise. This type of training can help to boost metabolism, burn calories, and improve cardiovascular fitness. For example, an endomorph senior could walk at a brisk pace for one minute, then slow down to a leisurely pace for two minutes, and repeat.

- Aim for at least 150 minutes of moderate-intensity cardio per week: The American Heart Association recommends that adults aim for at least 150 minutes of moderate-intensity cardio per week. This can be divided into several sessions throughout the week.

Cardiovascular exercise is an important component of any exercise program for endomorph seniors. It's important to choose low-impact exercises, monitor heart rate, and gradually increase intensity and duration over time. Working with a certified fitness trainer can help endomorph seniors design a safe and effective cardio program tailored to their individual needs and abilities

Chapter Five

ENDOMORPH BODY TYPE FOOD LIST

Comprehensive food list to eat

Proteins:

1. **Fish:**

   - Salmon

   - Mackerel

   - Sardines

   - Trout

2. **Lean Meats:**

   - Chicken breast

   - Turkey

   - Lean cuts of beef or pork

3. **Dairy:**

- Greek yogurt (low-fat or fat-free)

- Cottage cheese

- Eggs

4. **Plant-Based Proteins:**

   - Lentils

   - Chickpeas

   - Quinoa

   - Tofu

   - Edamame

5. **Nuts and Seeds:**

   - Almonds

   - Walnuts

   - Chia seeds

   - Flaxseeds

Vegetables:

1. **Leafy Greens:**

   - Spinach

   - Kale

   - Swiss chard

   - Collard greens

2. **Colorful Vegetables:**

   - Broccoli

   - Bell peppers

   - Carrots

   - Tomatoes

3. **Cruciferous Vegetables:**

   - Cauliflower

   - Brussels sprouts

   - Cabbage

4. **Root Vegetables:**

- Sweet potatoes

- Carrots

- Beets

5. **Legumes:**

- Beans (black beans, kidney beans, chickpeas)

- Lentils

Fruits:

1. **Berries:**

- Blueberries

- Strawberries

- Raspberries

2. **Citrus Fruits:**

  - Oranges

  - Grapefruits

  - Lemons

3. **Bananas**

4. **Apples**

5. **Avocado**

Whole Grains:

1. Quinoa

2. Brown rice

3. Oats

4. Barley

5. Whole grain bread and pasta

Healthy Fats:

1. Olive oil

2. Avocado

3. Nuts and seeds

4. Fatty fish (salmon, mackerel)

5. Flaxseed oil

Dairy or Dairy Alternatives:

1. Low-fat or fat-free milk

2. Low-fat or fat-free yogurt

3. Cheese in moderation

Fluids:

1. Water

2. Herbal teas

3. Low-sodium vegetable juice

Snacks:

1. Fresh fruit slices

2. Vegetable sticks with hummus

3. Greek yogurt with berries

4. Nuts and seeds mix

Herbs and Spices:

1. Turmeric

2. Cinnamon

3. Ginger

4. Garlic

5. Oregano

Supplements (as advised by a healthcare professional):

1. Calcium and Vitamin D for bone health

2. Omega-3 fatty acids

3. Multivitamins

Comprehensive list of foods to avoid

Processed and Sugary Foods:

1. Sodas and sugary drinks

2. Candy and sweets

3. Commercially baked goods (cakes, pastries, cookies)

4. Processed cereals with added sugars

Refined Carbohydrates:

1. White bread

2. White rice

3. White pasta

4. Refined breakfast cereals

Fried and Fast Foods:

1. French fries

2. Fried chicken

3. Fast food burgers and fries

4. Processed and fried snacks (potato chips, nachos)

High-Fat Meats:

1. Fatty cuts of red meat

2. Processed meats (sausages, hot dogs, bacon)

3. Fried and breaded meats

Full-Fat Dairy:

1. Full-fat milk

2. Full-fat cheese

3. Cream and butter in excess

High-Sugar and High-Fat Sauces:

1. Sweetened ketchup

2. Barbecue sauce with added sugars

3. Creamy and high-fat salad dressings

Highly Processed Snacks:

1. Packaged snacks with high sugar and fat content

2. Microwave popcorn with added butter

3. Processed cheese snacks

Alcohol:

1. Excessive alcohol consumption

2. Sweetened and high-calorie cocktails

Salty and High-Sodium Foods:

1. Processed and canned soups with high-sodium

2. Canned and processed meats

3. Excessively salty snacks (pretzels, salted nuts)

Sweetened and Flavored Beverages:

1. Sweetened fruit juices

2. Energy drinks

3. Flavored coffee drinks with added sugars

Artificial Sweeteners and Diet Products:

1. Diet sodas with artificial sweeteners

2. Sugar-free candies with artificial sweeteners

Highly Processed and Convenience Foods:

1. Frozen meals with high sodium and additives

2. Instant noodles and packaged convenience foods

3. Highly processed and pre-packaged meals

Considerations for Seniors:

1. Limit caffeine intake, especially in the evening.

2. Be cautious with spicy foods if they cause digestive discomfort.

3. Monitor portion sizes to avoid overeating.

Chapter Six

ENDOMORPH RECIPES

Grilled Chicken Salad

Ingredients:

4 oz grilled chicken breast

2 cups mixed greens

1/2 cup sliced cucumbers

1/2 cup cherry tomatoes

1/4 cup sliced red onion

2 tbsp olive oil

2 tbsp balsamic vinegar

Salt and pepper to taste

Instructions:

- Grill chicken breast until fully cooked.

- In a large bowl, combine mixed greens, cucumbers, cherry tomatoes, and red onion.

- Top the salad with the grilled chicken breast.
- Drizzle olive oil and balsamic vinegar over the salad.
- Season with salt and pepper to taste.

Nutritional Information (per serving):

Calories: 285

Protein: 28g

Carbohydrates: 10g

Fat: 16g

Quinoa and Black Bean Salad

Ingredients:

1 cup cooked quinoa

1 cup canned black beans, drained and rinsed

1/2 cup diced red bell pepper

1/2 cup diced green bell pepper

1/4 cup chopped fresh cilantro

2 tbsp olive oil

2 tbsp lime juice

Salt and pepper to taste

Instructions:

- In a large bowl, combine cooked quinoa, black beans, red and green bell peppers, and cilantro.

- In a small bowl, whisk together olive oil and lime juice.

- Drizzle the dressing over the quinoa and black bean salad.

- Season with salt and pepper to taste.

Nutritional Information (per serving):

Calories: 310

Protein: 12g

Carbohydrates: 38g

Fat: 12g

Baked Salmon with Roasted Vegetables

Ingredients:

4 oz salmon fillet

1 cup mixed vegetables (such as broccoli, carrots, and cauliflower)

2 tsp olive oil

Salt and pepper to taste

Instructions:

- Preheat oven to 375°F (190°C).

- Place the salmon fillet on a baking sheet lined with parchment paper.

- Toss mixed vegetables with olive oil and season with salt and pepper.

- Place the vegetables around the salmon fillet.

- Bake for 15-20 minutes, or until the salmon is fully cooked.

Nutritional Information (per serving):

Calories: 285

Protein: 28g

Carbohydrates: 10g

Fat: 16g

Turkey and Sweet Potato Skillet

Ingredients:

4 oz ground turkey

1/2 cup chopped sweet potato

1/4 cup chopped onion

1/4 cup chopped red bell pepper

1/2 tsp chili powder

Salt and pepper to taste

Instructions:

- In a large skillet, cook the ground turkey over medium-high heat until browned.

- Add chopped sweet potato, onion, and red bell pepper to the skillet.

- Season with chili powder, salt, and pepper.

- Cook for 10-12 minutes or until the sweet potato is tender.

Nutritional Information (per serving):

Calories: 230

Protein: 23g

Carbohydrates: 15g

Fat: 9g

Egg White Omelette with Spinach and Feta

Ingredients:

3 egg whites

1/2 cup fresh spinach

2 tbsp crumbled feta cheese

1/2 tsp olive oil

Salt and pepper to taste

Instructions:

• In a small bowl, whisk together egg whites.

• Heat olive oil in a non-stick skillet over medium heat.

- Add fresh spinach to the skillet and cook until wilted.

- Pour the egg whites into the skillet and cook until set.

- Sprinkle feta cheese on top of the omelette.

Fold the omelette in half and serve.

Nutritional Information (per serving):

Calories: 150

Protein: 20g

Carbohydrates: 2g

Fat: 6g

Turkey and Avocado Wrap

Ingredients:

4 oz sliced turkey breast

1/4 avocado, sliced

1 whole wheat wrap

1/4 cup sliced cucumber

1/4 cup sliced red onion

1/4 cup mixed greens

1 tsp honey mustard

Instructions:

- Lay the whole wheat wrap flat on a plate or cutting board.

- Spread honey mustard on the wrap.

- Layer sliced turkey, avocado, cucumber, red onion, and mixed greens on top of the honey mustard.

- Roll up the wrap tightly, tucking in the sides.

- Slice in half and serve.

Nutritional Information (per serving):

Calories: 280

Protein: 20g

Carbohydrates: 28g

Fat: 10g

Baked Sweet Potato Fries

Ingredients:

1 medium sweet potato, cut into fries

1 tbsp olive oil

1/2 tsp paprika

Salt and pepper to taste

Instructions:

- Preheat oven to 400°F (200°C).
- In a bowl, toss the sweet potato fries with olive oil, paprika, salt, and pepper.
- Spread the fries on a baking sheet lined with parchment paper.
- Bake for 20-25 minutes or until crispy and tender.

Nutritional Information (per serving):

Calories: 200

Protein: 2g

Carbohydrates: 29g

Fat: 9g

Quinoa and Sweet Potato Salad

Ingredients:

1 cup quinoa

1 large sweet potato, peeled and diced

1 red bell pepper, diced

1/2 red onion, diced

2 tablespoons olive oil

1 tablespoon honey

1 tablespoon Dijon mustard

1 tablespoon apple cider vinegar

Salt and pepper to taste

Instructions:

- Preheat the oven to 400°F (200°C).

- Cook the quinoa according to package instructions.

- Toss the diced sweet potato in 1 tablespoon of olive oil and season with salt and pepper. Roast in the oven for 20-25 minutes, until tender and lightly browned.

- In a small bowl, whisk together the remaining tablespoon of olive oil, honey, Dijon mustard, apple cider vinegar, salt, and pepper.

- In a large mixing bowl, combine the cooked quinoa, roasted sweet potato, diced red bell pepper, and diced red onion. Drizzle the dressing over the top and toss to combine.

Nutritional requirements:

Calories: 290

Protein: 6g

Fat: 10g

Carbohydrates: 44g

Fiber: 6g

Turkey and Vegetable Stir-Fry

Ingredients:

1 pound turkey breast, sliced

1 red bell pepper, sliced

1 yellow bell pepper, sliced

1 large carrot, sliced

1 small onion, sliced

2 cloves garlic, minced

2 tablespoons olive oil

2 tablespoons soy sauce

1 tablespoon honey

1 tablespoon cornstarch

1/4 cup water

Salt and pepper to taste

Instructions:

- In a large wok or skillet, heat the olive oil over medium-high heat.

- Add the sliced turkey breast and cook for 5-7 minutes, until browned on all sides.

- Add the sliced red and yellow bell peppers, sliced carrot, sliced onion, and minced garlic to the wok. Stir-fry for 5-7 minutes until the vegetables are tender-crisp.

- In a small bowl, whisk together the soy sauce, honey, cornstarch, water, salt, and pepper.

- Pour the sauce over the turkey and vegetables and stir-fry for another 2-3 minutes, until the sauce has thickened and the turkey and vegetables are coated.

Nutritional requirements:

Calories: 320

Protein: 32g

Fat: 9g

Carbohydrates: 26g

Fiber: 4g

Grilled Salmon with Roasted Vegetables

Ingredients:

4 salmon fillets

2 tablespoons olive oil

1 teaspoon garlic powder

1 teaspoon dried thyme

1 teaspoon dried oregano

Salt and pepper, to taste

2 cups mixed vegetables (such as broccoli, bell peppers, and onions)

1 tablespoon balsamic vinegar

1 tablespoon honey

1 tablespoon Dijon mustard

Instructions:

- Preheat the oven to 425°F (220°C).

- Arrange the mixed vegetables in a single layer on a baking sheet. Drizzle with 1 tablespoon of olive oil and sprinkle with garlic powder, salt, and pepper. Roast in the oven for 20-25 minutes, stirring once or twice, until tender and golden brown.

- While the vegetables are roasting, prepare the salmon. In a small bowl, mix the remaining olive oil, thyme, oregano, salt, and pepper.

• Brush the salmon fillets with the herb mixture and place them on a preheated grill or grill pan. Grill for 5-6 minutes on each side, until cooked through and slightly charred.

• In another small bowl, whisk together the balsamic vinegar, honey, and Dijon mustard.

• Serve the grilled salmon with the roasted vegetables and drizzle with the balsamic-honey-mustard sauce.

Nutritional Information:

Calories: 350

Fat: 20g

Carbohydrates: 11g

Fiber: 3g

Protein: 30g

Sodium: 280mg

Baked Chicken and Sweet Potato Mash

Ingredients:

4 boneless, skinless chicken breasts

2 tablespoons olive oil

2 teaspoons dried rosemary

Salt and pepper, to taste

4 medium sweet potatoes, peeled and chopped

1/4 cup unsweetened almond milk

1 tablespoon honey

1/2 teaspoon ground cinnamon

1/4 teaspoon ground nutmeg

Instructions:

- Preheat the oven to 400°F (200°C).
- Season the chicken breasts with olive oil, rosemary, salt, and pepper, and arrange them in a baking dish.

- Bake the chicken for 25-30 minutes, or until cooked through and no longer pink in the center.

- While the chicken is baking, place the sweet potatoes in a large pot and cover them with water. Bring to a boil over high heat, then reduce the heat to medium-low and simmer for 15-20 minutes, or until the sweet potatoes are soft and tender.

- Drain the sweet potatoes and return them to the pot. Add the almond milk, honey, cinnamon, nutmeg, salt, and pepper, and mash until smooth and creamy.

- Serve the baked chicken with a scoop of sweet potato mash.

Nutritional Information:
Calories: 350
Fat: 10g

Carbohydrates: 32g

Fiber: 5g

Protein: 35g

Sodium: 150mg

Quinoa Stuffed Peppers

Ingredients:

4 bell peppers, tops cut off and seeded

1 cup cooked quinoa

1/2 cup diced onion

1/2 cup diced mushrooms

1/2 cup diced zucchini

1/2 cup diced eggplant

1 clove garlic, minced

1 tablespoon olive oil

1 teaspoon dried oregano

Salt and pepper, to taste

1/4 cup grated Parmesan cheese

Instructions:

- Preheat the oven to 375°F (190°C).

- In a large skillet, heat the olive oil over medium-high heat. Add the onion, mushrooms, zucchini, eggplant, and garlic, and sauté for 5-7 minutes, or until the vegetables are tender.

- Stir in the cooked quinoa, oregano, salt, and pepper, and cook for an additional 2-3 minutes.

- Stuff the mixture into the bell peppers, packing it tightly. Sprinkle the Parmesan cheese over the top of the stuffed peppers.

- Place the stuffed peppers in a baking dish and bake for 30-35 minutes, or until the peppers are tender and the cheese is melted and bubbly.

Nutritional Information:

Calories: 200

Fat: 7g

Carbohydrates: 27g

Fiber: 7g

Protein: 9g

Sodium: 230mg

Grilled Chicken and Vegetable Kebabs

Ingredients:

1 lb boneless, skinless chicken breasts, cut into bite-sized pieces

1 red bell pepper, cut into bite-sized pieces

1 green bell pepper, cut into bite-sized pieces

1 yellow onion, cut into bite-sized pieces

1 zucchini, sliced

2 tablespoons olive oil

1 tablespoon chopped fresh rosemary

1 tablespoon chopped fresh thyme

1 tablespoon chopped fresh parsley

Salt and black pepper, to taste

Instructions:

- Preheat a grill to medium-high heat.

- Thread the chicken, bell peppers, onion, and zucchini onto skewers.

- In a small bowl, whisk together the olive oil, rosemary, thyme, parsley, salt, and black pepper.

- Brush the chicken and vegetables with the olive oil mixture.

- Grill the kebabs for 8-10 minutes, turning occasionally, or until the chicken is cooked through and the vegetables are tender.

Nutritional Information:

Calories: 260

Fat: 12g

Carbohydrates: 9g

Fiber: 3g

Protein: 30g

Sodium: 80mg

Greek Salad with Grilled Chicken

Ingredients:

1 lb. boneless, skinless chicken breasts

2 tbsp. olive oil

2 tbsp. red wine vinegar

1 tbsp. dried oregano

1 tsp. garlic powder

1 tsp. onion powder

Salt and pepper to taste

1 head romaine lettuce, chopped

1 cucumber, diced

1 red onion, sliced

1 pint cherry tomatoes, halved

1 cup kalamata olives, pitted

4 oz. feta cheese, crumbled

Instructions:

- Preheat the grill to medium-high heat.

- In a small bowl, whisk together olive oil, red wine vinegar, oregano, garlic powder, onion powder, salt, and pepper.

- Add chicken to a large bowl and pour marinade over the chicken. Toss to coat.

- Place chicken on the grill and cook for 5-6 minutes per side, or until internal temperature reaches 165°F. Let rest for 5 minutes before slicing.

- In a large bowl, add chopped romaine lettuce, diced cucumber, sliced red onion, halved cherry tomatoes, and pitted kalamata olives. Toss to combine.

- Divide salad mixture onto 4 plates, and top with sliced grilled chicken, and crumbled feta cheese.

- Serve and enjoy!

Nutritional information (per serving):

Calories: 408

Protein: 37g

Fat: 25g

Carbohydrates: 12g

Fiber: 4g

Quinoa and Black Bean Bowl

Ingredients:

1 cup quinoa, rinsed

2 cups water

1 tbsp. olive oil

1 onion, chopped

2 cloves garlic, minced

1 red bell pepper, chopped

1 tsp. chili powder

1/2 tsp. ground cumin

1/2 tsp. smoked paprika

1 can black beans, drained and rinsed

1/4 cup chopped fresh cilantro

Salt and pepper to taste

Lime wedges for serving

Instructions:

•   In a medium saucepan, combine quinoa and water. Bring to a boil, then reduce heat and simmer for 15-20 minutes, or until quinoa is tender and water is absorbed.

•   In a large skillet, heat olive oil over medium-high heat. Add chopped onion and minced garlic and sauté for 2-3 minutes, or until the onion is translucent.

•   Add chopped red bell pepper, chili powder, ground cumin, and smoked paprika to the skillet. Sauté for another 2-3 minutes, or until the red pepper is tender.

•   Add black beans to the skillet and stir to combine. Cook for another 2-3 minutes, or until beans are heated through.

- Add cooked quinoa to the skillet and stir to combine with the black bean mixture. Remove from heat and stir in chopped cilantro. Season with salt and pepper to taste.
- Divide the quinoa and black bean mixture into bowls and serve with lime wedges.

Nutritional information (per serving):

Calories: 330

Protein: 13g

Fat: 7g

Carbohydrates: 57g

Fiber: 13g

Mediterranean Tuna Salad

Ingredients:

2 cans of tuna, drained

1/4 cup diced red onion

1/4 cup diced cucumber

1/4 cup diced tomatoes

1/4 cup chopped Kalamata olives

1/4 cup crumbled feta cheese

2 tbsp. chopped fresh parsley

1 tbsp. extra-virgin olive oil

1 tbsp. lemon juice

Salt and pepper to taste

Instructions:

•	In a large bowl, combine the drained tuna, diced red onion, diced cucumber, diced tomatoes, chopped Kalamata olives, crumbled feta cheese, and chopped fresh parsley.

•	In a small bowl, whisk together the extra-virgin olive oil and lemon juice.

•	Pour the dressing over the tuna salad and toss to combine. Season with salt and pepper to taste.

- Serve the Mediterranean tuna salad chilled.

Nutritional information (per serving):

Calories: 310

Protein: 36g

Fat: 15g

Carbohydrates: 8g

Fiber: 2g

Broiled Salmon with Asparagus

Ingredients:

4 salmon fillets

1 bunch of asparagus

2 tbsp. olive oil

Salt and pepper to taste

1 lemon, sliced

Instructions:

- Preheat the broiler.

- Rinse the asparagus and trim the ends. Place the asparagus on a baking sheet and drizzle with 1 tablespoon of olive oil. Season with salt and pepper to taste.

- Place the salmon fillets on the baking sheet and brush with the remaining olive oil. Season with salt and pepper to taste.

- Place the lemon slices on top of the salmon fillets.

- Broil the salmon and asparagus for 8-10 minutes, or until the salmon is cooked through and the asparagus is tender.

- Serve the broiled salmon and asparagus immediately.

Nutritional information (per serving):

Calories: 360

Protein: 35g

Fat: 21g

Carbohydrates: 6g

Fiber: 2g

Grilled Salmon with Avocado Salsa

Ingredients:

4 salmon fillets

1 tablespoon olive oil

Salt and pepper, to taste

1 avocado, diced

1/4 cup red onion, diced

1/4 cup fresh cilantro, chopped

2 tablespoons lime juice

1 tablespoon olive oil

Instructions:

• Preheat the grill to medium-high heat.

• Brush the salmon fillets with olive oil and season with salt and pepper.

• Grill the salmon for 4-5 minutes per side, or until cooked through.

- While the salmon is grilling, prepare the avocado salsa. In a medium bowl, combine the diced avocado, red onion, cilantro, lime juice, and olive oil. Mix well.
- Serve the grilled salmon with a spoonful of the avocado salsa on top.

Nutritional Information:

Calories: 363

Fat: 22g

Protein: 34g

Carbohydrates: 8g

Fiber: 5g

Grilled Shrimp Skewers

Ingredients:

1 pound large shrimp, peeled and deveined

2 tablespoons olive oil

1 tablespoon fresh lemon juice

2 garlic cloves, minced

Salt and pepper, to taste

1 red bell pepper, cut into chunks

1 yellow onion, cut into chunks

8 wooden skewers, soaked in water for 30 minutes

Instructions:

• Preheat the grill to medium-high heat.

• In a large bowl, combine the shrimp, olive oil, lemon juice, garlic, salt, and pepper. Mix well.

• Thread the shrimp, red bell pepper, and onion onto the skewers.

• Grill the shrimp skewers for 2-3 minutes per side, or until the shrimp are pink and cooked through.

• Serve hot with your favorite dipping sauce.

Nutritional Information:

Calories: 173

Fat: 8g

Protein: 21g

Carbohydrates: 5g

Fiber: 1g

Roasted Vegetable and Chicken Quinoa Bowl

Ingredients:

1 pound boneless, skinless chicken breasts, diced

1 red onion, chopped

1 red bell pepper, chopped

1 yellow bell pepper, chopped

2 cups broccoli florets

2 cups cooked quinoa

2 tablespoons olive oil

1 teaspoon garlic powder

1 teaspoon paprika

Salt and pepper, to taste

Fresh parsley, chopped, for garnish

Instructions:

- Preheat the oven to 400°F (200°C).
- In a large bowl, toss the chicken, red onion, red and yellow bell peppers, and broccoli with olive oil, garlic powder, paprika, salt, and pepper.
- Spread the mixture out on a baking sheet and roast for 20-25 minutes, or until the chicken is cooked through and the vegetables are tender.
- To assemble the bowls, divide the cooked quinoa among four bowls.
- Top the quinoa with the roasted chicken and vegetable mixture.
- Garnish with chopped parsley.

Nutritional information:

Calories: 380

Fat: 12g

Carbohydrates: 35g

Fiber: 7g

Protein: 33g

Chapter Seven

CONCLUSION

In conclusion, crafting a thoughtful and tailored diet for seniors with an endomorphic body type is a vital step toward promoting their overall health and well-being. Understanding the unique characteristics and challenges associated with the endomorphic physique allows for the development of a comprehensive food list that caters to their specific needs.

The emphasis on a diet rich in lean proteins, such as chicken, turkey, and fish, provides essential nutrients for muscle maintenance, ultimately aiding in the optimization of metabolism. Simultaneously, the inclusion of plant-based proteins like lentils and tofu ensures a well-rounded nutritional profile, supporting seniors in achieving their health goals.

Careful consideration of carbohydrate intake, favoring whole grains, fruits, and vegetables, helps manage blood sugar levels and mitigates the risk of weight gain. By incorporating complex carbohydrates into their diet, seniors can enjoy sustained energy levels and a reduced likelihood of developing chronic conditions like diabetes.

Balancing fat consumption with a focus on healthy sources like nuts, seeds, and avocados contributes to an optimal caloric intake. The integration of omega-3 fatty acids from fatty fish, such as salmon, fosters heart health and aids in weight management.

Portion control emerges as a pivotal aspect of the endomorph diet for seniors, given their slower metabolism. Smaller, more frequent meals not only satisfy hunger but also prevent overeating, ensuring a sustainable approach to weight management.

Hydration remains a cornerstone of this dietary approach, as it aids in appetite control and supports weight loss. Encouraging seniors to maintain adequate fluid intake, primarily through water, fosters overall health and well-being.

Complementing this well-structured diet is the imperative inclusion of regular exercise, encompassing both strength training and cardiovascular activities. The synergy between proper nutrition and physical activity holds the key to building and maintaining muscle mass, enhancing metabolism, and fostering a healthier lifestyle for seniors.

In navigating the complexities of the endomorph body type, seniors need to seek personalized guidance from healthcare professionals or registered dietitians. This ensures that dietary recommendations align with individual health needs, promoting sustained success and an active, fulfilling life for seniors with an endomorphic body type.